ZEOLITE

Improve Your Health with Nature's Cleanser and Detoxifier

Dr. Howard Peiper N.D.

ZEOLITE

by

Dr. Howard Peiper

All Rights Reserved

Printed in the U.S.A.
First Printing, October 2006
Revised Edition, May 2012
Updated Printing, January 2020

Published by
WTP Publications
(760) 902-3343

Table of Contents

Author's Statement

I believe we need to be aware of the potentially tragic and harmful effects of the numerous chemicals, which assault our bodies on a daily basis.

This booklet will discuss the many different ways chemicals can affect you and your loved ones. Do not feel overwhelmed, but rather feel empowered and recognize that practical sensible answers do exist with many being inexpensive, easy and effective. Prevention and avoidance are the keys. Detoxification and elimination of chemicals from your body is a necessity! You can truly turn your life around. Your present health can improve and your future well being can be made much more secure.

Howard Peiper, N.D.

Chemicals and Pesticides Can Hurt You and Those You Love

Is it necessary to be afraid? Maybe. Industry data from the EPA (Environmental Protection Agency) indicates that 3.9 billion pounds of chemical that potentially can be harmful to humans were released into the air and water nationwide in 2017. There are over 86,000 chemicals presently used in the United States. Less than nine percent of these chemicals in relation to healthy young males have been properly studied for their effects on the human immune, nervous, endocrine and reproductive systems.

The facts are that chemicals can be a problem for anyone, at any age. Their safety has never been checked as to their effects on the unborn, young children, females, pregnant women or older individuals who are the most apt to have adverse effects. Even at risk is anyone who has a depressed immune system, such as a cancer patient undergoing chemotherapy. Almost any area of the body can be vulnerable and can be adversely affected from chemicals or other harmful environmental exposures. Sensitivities to chemicals can begin at any time. Therefore, for those who think of themselves as immune to chemicals, they had better get educated before it's too late.

Over 900 different types of chemicals, such as herbicides, insecticides, termiticides or fungicides are collectively called pesticides. Of the 63 active pesticides used in schools, statistics show: 18 are probable causes of cancer, 24 are related to birth defects, 45 appear to cause reproduction problems, 48 can affect the central nervous system, 54 can damage the kidneys and 60 may cause eye and skin problems.

Is it necessary to be afraid? Maybe. Better succumbing to fear, let this booklet empower you by giving you the knowledge you need to help and protect yourself!

Industrial Toxins

A great number of highly toxic chemicals, materials, and heavy metals are released by industrial processes and find their way into the human body. Heavy metals, such as lead, arsenic, mercury, aluminum, nickel, cadmium, and many others have no safe level in the human system. These toxins may accumulate within the fat cells, central nervous system, bones, brain, glands, or hair, and manifest negative health effects.

The claim that environmental chemicals can cause or promote cancer is supported by the fact that the distribution of toxic-waste dump sites closely correlates with those locations being synonymous with high rates of breast cancer mortality, according to *Scientific American* (October 1995). A variety of chemicals found in the environment can mimic the activity of estrogen once inside the human body; and are now believed to contribute to many cases of breast cancer. By 1983, the EPA had detected over 420 toxic chemicals in human tissue; 48 in fat tissue, 42 in breast milk, 75 in the liver, and 252 in the blood.

Industrial workers are routinely exposed to potentially toxic chemicals and substances while on the job. Tanners, oil refinery workers, and insecticide/herbicide sprayers are exposed to arsenic and risk lung and skin cancer. Shipyard workers, demolition experts, and brake mechanics are exposed to asbestos, which place them at risk for lung cancer. Hospital and laboratory staffs, as well as those involved in the manufacture of wood products are routinely exposed to formaldehyde. School biology labs using formaldehyde in their petri dishes can affect students. Even that new car smell every one associates with luxury is in many cases formaldehyde outgassing from seat and carpet fabric.

Other carcinogens in the workplace, such as benzene, diesel exhaust, human-made fibers, hair dyes, mineral oils, painting materials, polychlorinated biphenyl, and soot, are linked with specific occupations, routine exposures, and various cancers (*Atlantic Monthly* June 1996). It is estimated that 12 percent of all cancers are attributable to job related exposures to carcinogens (*Radiology* 178, 1991).

Polluted Water

Tap water is becoming a health hazard in the U.S. It is not just pesticides and agricultural runoffs that contaminate public drinking water, but according to the EPA, the tap water of 30 million Americans contains potentially hazardous levels of lead (*National Women's Health Network,* 1993). In addition, one out of every three public water systems have violated federal standards for tap water. Municipal water can contain many different contaminants, including disease-causing bacteria, radioactive particles, heavy metals, gasoline solvents, industrial wastes, chemical residues, and synthetic organic chemicals.

More recently, the 2015 Flint, Michigan lead emergency highlighted the dangers lurking in our municipal water systems, as the community was left fighting for clean water. A 2017 report from the Natural Resources Defense Council indicated that in 2015 alone, nearly 77 million people were served from municipal water systems that violated health protective safety standards. In addition, CDC has reported that over 19 million people in the US fall ill every year as a result of pathogens found in contaminated drinking water from public water systems. Past studies have revealed that many municipal water systems contain significant levels of arsenic, radon, and chlorine by-products and that hundreds of major water suppliers and agencies fail to give consumers information on their tap water. Polluted drinking water can further raise the risk of developing cancer.

Mercury Toxicity

Mercury, a toxic heavy metal that often comprises up to 51 percent of "silver amalgam" dental fillings, is a noted carcinogen and has the ability to impair immune function and create blockages in the autonomic nervous system and other tissues. Evidence now shows that mercury amalgams are the major source of mercury exposure for the general public, at rates six times higher than that found in seafood.

Since mercury vapors are continuously released from amalgam fillings, as long as you have those type of dental fillings in your mouth, you inhale mercury vapor 24 hours a day and 365 days a year. After elemental mercury from amalgam fillings is inhaled or ingested it is converted in the body to methyl-mercury, the organic form of mercury. Methyl-mercury, because it easily crosses the blood-brain barrier has been associated with neurodegenerative diseases such as Alzheimer's, Multiple Sclerosis, and amyotrophic lateral sclerosis. As toxic as elemental mercury is, methyl-mercury is 120 times more toxic. The *New England Journal of Medicine*, 2003;349 (18) pointed out that "the fetal brain is more susceptible than the adult brain to mercury induced damage". Specifically, methyl-mercury "inhibits the division and migration of neuronal cells and disrupts the cytoarchitecture of the developing brain". Recent studies have correlated the explosive increase of autism with thimerosal, an additive to many vaccines that contains 54% percent ethyl mercury.

Mercury is a heavy metal. Heavy metals act as free radicals – highly reactive, charged particles that can cause damage to body tissues. Like other heavy metals, mercury has been shown to cause damage to the lining of arteries and nerve bundles (ganglia), particularly those near the prostate.

The EPA recently reported that a third of the country's lakes and nearly a quarter of its rivers are now so polluted with mercury that children and pregnant women are advised to limit or avoid eating fish caught there. Warnings about mercury, a highly toxic metal used in things ranging from dental fillings to watch batteries have been issued by 45 states and cover four of the five Great Lakes. Mining, waste incineration and coal combustion convert it into methyl-mercury, a compound that works its way up the food chain into fish and eventually humans.

Nuclear Radiation

Working or living in the proximity of nuclear power plants presents a cancer risk. Among the hazards are the small amounts of radioactive gases released daily from nuclear reactors at levels deemed "permissible" by the U.S. Department of Energy. This low-level radioactive pollution returns to us in rainfall, which then accumulates in the soil to contaminate the food chain. People who eat dairy products and other foods tainted by these radioactive releases may be unwittingly exposing themselves to dangerous carcinogens. Since dairy products tend to concentrate the radioactive fission products avoiding such foods may lower your cancer risk

According to Ernest Sternglass, Ph.D., Professor of Radiation Physics at Univ. of Pittsburgh, "Chronic exposure to nuclear fission products through the diet and drinking water may be the single largest factor in the increased incidence of most forms of malignancies since 1945."

Other Common Toxic Chemicals Found In Humans:

DIOXINS (by-products of PVC production, industrial bleaching and incineration): Dioxins are known to cause cancer in animals, and there is some concern that even low-level exposure over long periods of time can disrupt normal functioning of the endocrine (hormone) system, resulting in reproductive or developmental effects.

FURANS (pollutants, by-products of plastic production): Furans cause cancer in humans and are toxic to endocrine system.

PHTHALATES (found in many cosmetics and personal care products): Phthalates cause birth defects in male reproductive organs.

PCBs (industrial insulators and lubricants): PCBs were banned in the U.S. in 1076 due to their connection to increased cancer rates and central nervous system disorder.

How Often Does Exposure to Toxic Chemicals Cause Illness?

It is estimated that over 12 million Americans are so severely affected by toxic chemicals that they must totally change their lifestyle and no longer can live in a normal manner.

Toxic chemicals in humans have been reported to alter:

- normal development of the unborn leading to miscarriages, stillbirths, birth anomalies and delays in normal development. *(At least 3 million children presently suffer from developmental, learning and behavioral difficulties.)*

- the immune system causing an increased tendency to allergies and recurrent respiratory (nose, sinus or lung) or ear infections.

- defense systems of human bodies making them more prone to cancer.

- our brain and nervous system causing headaches, difficulty thinking or remembering, inexplicable emotional ups and downs, inconsolable depression, irritability, moodiness, aggression, hyperactivity or extreme fatigue.

- the endocrine system, contributing to illnesses such as diabetes, thyroid disease and weakened adrenal glands.

- our reproductive system causing a wide variety of sexual problems and infertility.

- muscular system causing twitches, tics, muscle pain or weakness, in time possibly leading to Fibromyalgia, MS, amyotrophic lateral sclerosis or Parkinson's disease.

- skeletal system causing chronic swelling and stiffness that eventually leads to pain and permanent joint deformities.

- heart and circulatory system causing high blood pressure or irregular heartbeats.

- blood vessels causing abnormal bleeding into the skin, joints, breasts, urine and elsewhere.

There is a Solution!

Zeolite. Millions of years ago, zeolite deposits formed when volcanoes erupted enormous amounts of ash-aluminosilicates of alkaline and alkaline earths. Some of the wind borne ash settled to form thick ash beds. In some cases the ash fell into lakes and in others water percolated through the ash beds. In all cases, the chemical reaction of volcanic ash and salt water resulted in the formation of natural zeolites.

The characteristics of a zeolite deposit are decided in its genesis. Small natural differences such as temperature, geographic location and ash/water properties impart a slightly different composition and therefore, some unique properties to a few of the deposits. These small differences present during the formation of a zeolite deposit are the reason that each natural zeolite property has distinctly unique properties.

The alumina and silica from the ash stack into a stable, open and three-dimensional honey comb structure, there are over forty other natural zeolite structures. For example, clinoptilolite (a member of the zeolite group of minerals) has silica to alumina ratio of four to one.

Zeolite is an amazing crystalline mineral capable of adsorbing and absorbing many different types of gases, moisture, petrochemicals, heavy metals, low-level radioactive elements and a multitude of various solutions. The channels in the zeolite provide large surface areas on which chemical reactions can take place. The cavities and channels within the crystal could occupy up to 51 percent of its volume. Zeolites can adsorb or absorb large amounts of material such as ions or gas molecules.

There are three main kinds of zeolite: fibrous, leafy or crystalline. Medical use is from crystalline zeolite that contains high quantities of the mineral clinoptilolite.

How Does It Work?

It's extremely hard, micro-porous, honeycomb type of structure is permeated by ducts and cavities throughout. These caves or channels are openings where either minerals or heavy metals can bind. The silicon building block is electrically neutral, but the aluminum building block carries a negative charge creating charged sites throughout the entire crystal structure. The balancing process that works to maintain electroneutrality in the clinoptilolite attracts positive minerals such as calcium, magnesium, potassium, sodium and iron. These common cations (positively charged ions) can easily be displaced by heavy metals such as cadmium, mercury, nickel, and arsenic and be removed from the body.

Zeolite has a history of industrial and veterinary use, including water purification, air filters, in animal feed to reduce the production of ammonia and increase the nutritive effect, and in cat litter and animal stalls to reduce odor. It has even been put in cigarette filters to reduce nicotine and tar.

Medical Uses of Zeolite

Zeolite As An Anti-Diarrheal

Many people chronically suffer from abdominal cramps and bloating, they also may suffer from diarrhea and constipation. These symptoms may be the result of Irritable Bowel Syndrome (IBS). IBS is the term used to describe the situation in which the digestive tract is not functioning, as it should.

It is estimated between 21-51 million Americans have IBS, and this condition accounts for 2-3 visits to the doctor annually. Although IBS affects people of all ages, races and genders, nearly two-thirds are females.

Natural silicate materials have been shown to exhibit diverse biological activities and have been used successfully as a vaccine adjuvant and for the treatment of diarrhea and IBS.

The potential growth promoting action of natural zeolites has been attributed to their high affinity for ammonium ions, resulting to the reduction in the uptake of ammonia produced from deamination of proteins during digestive processes via the intestinal wall. Ammonia is recognized as a cell toxicant and the reduction of the amount, which the intestinal epithelial cells are exposed to, could lead to a reduction of epithelial turnover, sparing of energy and a better nutrient utilization.

The best-known, positive activity of natural zeolite is its action as an anti-diarrheal product. Zeolites lower the incidence of death and sickness produced by intestinal diseases in various animals. Based on these results a comprehensive study (Rodriguez-Fuentes 1997) was carried out on anti-diarrheal drugs based on natural zeolite as an active material, in the therapy of acute diarrheal diseases in humans. The research led to approval of the anti-diarrheal drug Enterex for use in humans.

Ingestion of zeolites may be considered analogous to clay eating, considered in traditional medicine as a remedy for various illnesses. The bulk of ingested zeolite remains undissolved in the gut. Because of the ion exchange properties, zeolites can change the ionic content, pH, and buffering capacity of the gastrointestinal secretions and to affect the transport through the intestinal epithelium. Also, zeolites can affect the bacterial flora and the resorption of vitamins and minerals. The contact of zeolite particles with gastrointestinal mucosa may elicit the secretion of cytokines (a part of our immune system) with local and systemic actions. This creates a healthier digestive tract with beneficial flora and fauna.

A zeolite product that I would recommend is Esdifan capsules by ZEO Health.

Zeolite And Mycotoxins

Zeolite is known to bind a range of mycotoxins, forming highly stable complexes (Tomasevic-Canovic and Huwig 2001). Mycotoxins are a diverse family of toxins produced by certain fungi especially by species of Aspergillus, Claviceps and Alternaria. There are several hundred distinct mycotoxins, capable of causing health problems such as renal and hepatic syndromes and diminished immune system. The most extensively researched mycotoxins are the aflatoxins (i.e. found in corn, peanuts, milk and cereals), which have been linked to liver, stomach, and kidney cancer. The ability of zeolite to adsorb the aflatoxins has resulted in measurable improvements in the health of various animals (Mumpton, Pariat 1999 and Kyriakis 2002).

Zeolite As A Heavy Metal Adsorbent

Many toxic heavy metals have been discharged into the environment as industrial wastes, causing serious soil and water pollution. The main threats to human health are exposure to mercury, cadmium, lead, and arsenic. These metals have been extensively studied and their effects on human health regularly reviewed by international bodies such as WHO (World Health Organization, 1993).

Studies have shown that zeolite has a high affinity for trapping lead, cadmium, arsenic, mercury and other potentially harmful metals. Through the process of cation exchange, zeolite can lower overall heavy metal exposure in individuals. This would have a dramatic effect in the risk reduction of certain cancers and heart disease.

What is very interesting is that zeolite appears to remove toxins in a certain order. It first removes the above heavy metals within the first few weeks, then it removes secondary priority toxins, including pesticides, herbicides and plastics.

Author's note: *" I have been taking Zeolite Pure Powder (ZEO Health) for years and have noticed constant improvements in mental clarity, increased energy and a continued sense of peace and well-being."*

Zeolite and pH

The scale used to measure the body's acidity and alkalinity is called pH, normally measured in a range from one to fourteen. A neutral solution nether acidic nor alkaline, has a pH of seven; acid is less than seven, alkaline is more than seven. The blood must be kept within the very narrow range of pH 7.4 to maintain homeostasis (balance).

Unfortunately, the average North American diet is very high in acid foods, such as sugar, refined carbohydrates and starch. These are not conductive to maintaining proper pH balance in the body and raise acid levels. To prevent disease from getting a foothold in this acid environment it is imperative that homeostasis be restored.

The body has a wide array of mechanisms to maintain homeostasis in the blood and extracellular fluid. The most important way that the pH of the blood is kept relatively constant is by buffers dissolved in the blood.

Zeolite buffers the system towards slight alkalinity by establishing pH levels of 7.35 - 7.45, which is the optimum pH for the human body. The body's pH level influences both immunity and brain function.

An acid blood pH (7.34 or lower) creates a precondition for cancer. In an acid environment, brain cell function can also be impaired, causing depression, anxiety, stupor, paranoia, delusions or hallucinations.

Zeolite as a Potent Antioxidant

Over 90 percent of different diseases (malignant, cardiovascular, diabetes, arthritis, neurodegenerative etc,) and aging, appear as the consequences of cellular functional disorder and the damage of the cell itself caused by direct or indirect influence of Oxygen Free Radicals. Free radicals supervise many processes in transmission of signals and expression of genes.

Smoking, incorrect eating habits, different radiation and exposure to harmful chemicals decrease natural defensive power of an organism and increase the danger of free radical damage. For example, scientific studies have shown that people who smoke have 30-45 times more damage to their DNA than non-smokers. Therefore, cells and tissues are constantly exposed to the affects of oxygen radicals.

With its own antioxidant system the cell protects itself from free radical damage. But over time that defensive system weakens and when under the influence of free radicals, becomes insufficient resulting in damage to the cell.

Zeolite is a unique antioxidant. A traditional antioxidant works by absorbing excess free radicals into its system because it has an unpaired electron. In contrast, zeolite traps free radicals in its complex structure, inactivating and eliminating them.

Zeolite and Cancer

The development of modern industry has caused increasingly serious pollution in the environment constituting a catastrophic health risk, including cancer. Cancer prevention is thus one of the challenges facing scientists in the twenty-first century, and removal of carcinogens from the environment is an important step.

Nitrosamines are probably the most widespread carcinogens, existing in the workplace, processed meats, cigarette smoke and beer. Many carcinogenic agents like nitrosamines or their precursors enter the human stomach through diet and drinking. Environmental pollution makes this hidden trouble more serious, because of the contaminated food and polluted atmosphere. However, although nitrosamines are well known carcinogenic substances, they require metabolic activation before reaction with DNA to cause mutation and cancer. It is very possible and necessary to trap the nitrosamines in the digestive tract provided a selective adsorbent material is used. Zeolite is considered as the best candidate. Zeolite has been used in slow released drugs, enzyme mimetic drugs, anti-tumor drugs and additives in cigarettes to remove carcinogenic agents like nitrosamines.

In summary, zeolite's mechanism of action against cancer cells is unique and unlike that of any other substance. It has the rare ability to take in a tremendous amount of positively charged toxins, indirectly neutralizing their effect in causing cancer. In the process, the zeolite develops a slight positive charge. It then attracted to and pulled right into the negatively charged membrane of the cancer cell. When the zeolite moves into the cancer cell, the cell's P21 gene is activated. This gene acts as a tumor suppressor through its ability to control cell-cycle progression. The activation of P21 halts the growth of tumors by indirectly suppressing growth signals.

Zeolite and Viruses

The list of diseases caused by viruses is immense and range from the common cold to cancer. Viruses not only cause specific diseases with clear diagnostic symptoms, but can also cause a constellation of symptoms that can defy diagnosis. Some viral diseases mimic other illness (for example, fatigue caused by anemia), or secondary inflammation (joint pain associated with arthritis). Certain viruses have specific affinity for only one type of tissue such as the liver or skin, while others an attraction to the body organs and systems. Viruses can cause localized infections such as warts or a sore throat, or a generalized infection such as in influenza, in which your whole body feels sick.

Zeolite has the capability to trap pre-virus components, preventing the replication of viruses and their ability to cause various conditions. Zeolite absorbs viral parts into the pores of the micronized zeolite aggregates This is the reason why zeolite seems to block the development of many viral infections, including herpes virus 1, Coxsackie virus B-5, and adenovirus 5. There have been many studies in cases of herpes zoster patients that have become pain free within one to three days after beginning to take zeolite. Other studies have shown that it is effective in treating the flu, colds, hepatitis C, viral or heavy metal induced multiple sclerosis, and rheumatoid arthritis. It also helps liver enzymes (AST, ALT) in reaching normal values.

Zeolite's effect as an anti-viral appears to be a preventative function that builds up over time, beginning after approximately four to six weeks of use, when heavy metals, pesticides, and herbicides have been mostly eliminated. There is anecdotal evidence, however, that in some cases its antiviral effect seems to be immediate.

Zeolite and the Immune System

The immune system's basic function is to protect us against infection, illness and disease of all kinds. It fights off thousands of predatory environmental and infectious microorganisms, which can invade and damage virtually every part of the body. The immune system has the ability to expel pathogens (virus, bacteria, etc.), toxic chemicals and tumorous cells that are generated through mutation. It also aids the body in tissue repair and healing and strives to maintain homeostasis (balance) in the body.

Zeolite appears to balance the immune system and   because it so powerfully removes various types of toxins from the body it naturally increases energy, well-being, and mental clarity. These are what we term positive secondary effects. Clearing out heavy metals allows the body's magnesium stores to work efficiently with adenosine triphosphate (ATP), the biological source of energy in the body. When this interaction is occurring optimally, people have more energy and experience greater well-being One study showed that zeolite also appears to increase serotonin level, which is known to help alleviate some forms of depression.

Zeolite and Hangovers

Alcohol intoxication causes dehydration and an imbalance in electrolytes, minerals and some vitamins in the bloodstream disrupting many normal biological processes. Additionally, when the blood alcohol is high, liver enzymes responsible for detoxification cannot function quickly enough so that toxic metabolites are produced. Such metabolites may be more toxic than alcohol and can cause nausea, headaches, and discomfort, usually referred to as a "hangover." Congeners, toxic byproducts of distillation and fermentation, worsen hangovers. Some alcoholic beverages such as red wine, brandies, and whiskies have higher concentration of congeners than others. Zeolite relieves the deleterious side effects of excessive alcohol consumption.

Zeolite's Effect on Other Conditions

Throughout this booklet, I have informed you about the way zeolite can benefit your body's most critical physiological system. From detoxifying toxic chemicals from the body, to providing your immune system with the necessary firepower to combat infections, zeolite is emerging as one of human kind's most beneficial allies.

Below is a list of other various diseases that can be treated by taking zeolite:

- *Circulatory system*: stabilization of the circulatory system along with improved blood pressure and reduced varicosity of the veins, reduction of and complete recovery from edema, swollen veins, hemorrhoids and disappearance of enlarged capillaries. Strengthening of the heart muscle, acceleration of post heart attack recuperation.

- *Rheumatic Disorders*: improved treatment of all types of rheumatic disorders, including sciatica, discopathy, arthritis, spondilosis, and rheumatic arthritis.

- *Kidney Function*: diuretic effect and positive influence in improving kidney function and treatment of kidney infection.

- *Skin Diseases*: treatment of skin diseases such as seborrhea, dermatitis, herpes (all types), psoriasis, and others, through either oral intake and/or external application of powder.

- *Diabetes Mellitus*: stabilization and decrease in the level of sugar in the blood.

- *Endocrine Glands*: optimization of endocrine gland activity, especially in the lymph nodes.

- *Wounds and Burns*: accelerated healing of wounds by direct application of powder. Also, direct application of powder to minor burns relieves pain and eliminates skin damage.

- *Periodontosis*: treatment of periodontosis and elimination of micro-organisms in the mouth with powder applied directly to the gums or as an additive to toothpaste.

- *Improving Skin Quality*: increased moisture, as well as significantly increasing resistance to various negative external factors including UV rays.

- *Neuro-psychiatric Effects*: overall improvement of disposition, successful treatment of insomnia, neurosis, and depression. Aids in the treatment of epilepsy, schizophrenia, Alzheimer's disease and Parkinson's disease.

- *Increasing Endurance:* increased endurance in situations of increased physical effort, reduction or elimination of pain resulting from increased physical exertion.

- *Fungal Infection*: quick and complete elimination of various fungal infections of the skin (Candida and others) and mucous membrane with direct application of powder. Elimination of fungal foot infections and treatment of fungal infections on internal organs, which can result from radiological procedures in combination with antibiotics.

To see improvements in any of these discussed ailments and conditions, it is important to use the purest zeolite source possible. ZEO Health has proved time and again that they provide the purest, most potent zeolite available.

Zeolite for Athletes

Clinical studies and sports scientific research have shown that activated zeolite in athletes affects the reduction of the percentage of lactate, reduction of free radicals, quick regeneration, increased sustainability, visibly better success at competitions and overall betterment of the total physical condition of athletes.

Zeolite powder contributes to the increase of sustainability of the body in terms of increased physical effort, as well as reduction and elimination of muscular   pain resulting from increased strain, which is particularly important for all athletes.

Zeolite for athletes particularly provides the following:

- reduction of free radicals
- reduction of the percentage of lactate
- faster regeneration
- visible better success at competitions

One recent study on 24 active athletes taken 5 grams of zeolite powder daily for 30 days, proved the ability of zeolite to reduce lactate. The athletes had increased efficiency by 13.98% on average, and maximally by 26% (at level 2 mmol/l lactate), confirming the unique ability of zeolite. (Lactate Study 2004, Knapitsch & Schmolzer)

The results of the study indicated that zeolite lowers the level of lactic acid that is responsible for the failing of the muscles in exercise. Alkalinity of zeolite lowers the lactic acid which in turn increases stamina and longevity in physical activity.

Regular intake of zeolite powder, acts on the entire detoxification of the body from heavy metals, ammonia, and an entire spectrum of dangerous toxins that threaten the health and vitality of humans. It prevents stress and numerous health problems, so it is recommended not only to athletes, but to all people with active lifestyles and those that are exposed to increased daily stress.

Zeolite is a valuable ally in slimming diets. Diets that lead to rapid weight loss cause a condition in the body called toxicity, because under normal conditions lipophilic toxins, such as dioxins, are stored in body fat and released and excreted slowly but steadily. If one loses large amounts of fat abruptly then huge amounts of lipophilic toxins are released into the body with serious health implications. Therefore, before anyone begins their weight loss quest, make sure to start taking zeolite powder to dispose of harmful substances from the body, and to lose weight safely.

Zeolite for Pets

Recently the U.S. Food and Drug Administration (FDA) reported that dog and cat food was released containing aflatoxin, a naturally occurring toxic chemical that comes from a fungus found in corn and other grains that causes severe liver damage in animals.

Animals that ingested food containing this toxic mold suffered permanent liver damage, which literally has killed many pets. Owners of these animals suffer emotionally and financially. Over 100 dogs have died so far from this toxin, leaving many more severely sick.

A study was conducted on aflatoxins found in grains fed to chickens. Researchers found that aflatoxins caused unfavorable microscopic changes to the liver, kidney, spleen, reproductive organs, and increased susceptibility to some environmental and uctive infectious agents. These are the same aflatoxins that are being accidentally fed our dogs and cats.

The study concluded that the powdered form of zeolite has the ability to absorb the aflatoxins, which resulted in measurable improvements in the health of various animals.

Natural zeolite has been shown to exhibit diverse biological activities and has been used successfully as a vaccine adjuvant and for the treatment of diarrhea in animals. The use of finely micronized zeolite as a treatment for dogs and cats suffering from a variety of tumors led to improvement in the animals' overall health statuses, prolongation of life-spans, and decreased tumor sizes. Local application of zeolite (powdered) to skin cancers of the animals effectively reduced tumor formation and growth.

In addition, toxicology studies showed that the treatment did not have negative effects.

In vitro tissue culture studies showed that finely micronized zeolite inhibits protein kinase B (c-Akt) and blocks cell growth in several cancer cell lines. (Bedrica, Hadzija 2001)

Liquid vs. Powder

There are two different types of liquid zeolites on the market. You should know that zeolites are a volcanic mineral and made up of compounds. It is important that the compound remains intact to be considered a zeolite and is what makes it so effective and beneficial for health. One type of liquid zeolite being sold is where they are using marketing gimmick names like "hydrolyzed" or "activated". You should understand that this whole liquid zeolite movement was a multilevel marketing company wanting to have something unique to build distributors and make money. The original attempt was using a process where the zeolite is exposed to hydrochloric acid and is broken down in a reaction chamber. The inventor never claimed it was a zeolite any longer after the process. The original intent was to create a injectable cancer drug. The MLM company who started this movement and licensed the process, found it difficult to do this process and it didn't work properly. They ended up just putting small amounts of micronized zeolite powder in water and calling it a liquid zeolite (the second type of liquid zeolite sold on the market today). The MLM company was eventually sued by their own distributors because the amount of zeolite in the product was less than 10% of the amount claimed and it was only 60% purity.

Synthetic Zeolites

There have been a few other companies who have tried to copy the original liquefying process and those products are on the market today. Once you destroy the cage structure of the zeolite and essentially the compound, you have a synthetic product and what could be considered a drug since it is no longer natural. There are other types of synthetic zeolites which should never be used for human consumption and were created by Mobil in the 1970's to be used for oil spills and toxic clean ups. One of those types is called Zeolite-A. There are many others.

Nano Zeolite

Some of these marketing gimmicks with the liquids are saying that their zeolites are nano size particles and so frustratingly ridiculous once you understand why. Zeolites work by using their negative charge to attract the toxins and heavy metals to the zeolite and trapping them in the zeolite cage so the body isn't re-exposed to the heavy metals, (which is why detox with zeolite has very little side effects). Nano particles make no sense because it is against the laws of physics. How can a particle smaller than the heavy metal particle, pick it up and carry it out of the body? It can't. That would be like trying to carry a building away in a bus. It just doesn't make sense. But these companies count on the internet to create hype and confusing consumers so they can make money on what is essentially a very expensive tiny bottle of water filled with the remnants of an acid wash of a zeolite.

There is a product called Zetox liquid suspension (Regal Supplements) that I recommend that has the highest amount of any micronized zeolite in a mix of complimentary vitamins that is perfect to be used as an introduction to zeolite detoxing, for use with children (it tastes good), maintenance detox, or as a temporary convenience for travel.

Those people who need therapeutic dosing and heavy detox, should stick with a micronized Clinoptilolite powder product such as Zeolite Pure powder (ZEO Health, the company that pioneered zeolite supplementation over 20 years ago).

Clinical Studies

Zeolite Influencing The Cellular Signal Transduction Pathways

"Clinical observations suggest that zeolite may be particularly promising in tumors known to respond to immune treatment with interferons and interleukins, like melanoma, renal cell cancer, lung cancer, and grade II and III astrocytoma. Significant improvements have been seen in 39 lung cancer patients and in 21 individuals suffering from glioblastoma (tumor of the central nervous system) after a three-week treatment with 12-16 grams of zeolite daily. Some patients with melanoma stage III and IV or lung cancer survived relapse-free for up to 6 years, respectively, on a long-term treatment."

Dr.s S. Ivkovic, T. Baranel, P. Bendzko and J. Schulz, Croatia 1998

Zeolite-Based Anti-Diarrheic Medication Approved By The Cuban Drug Control Agency

Four clinical studies were conducted using a zeolite-based anti-diarrheic medication.

In the first study, 18 men and 15 women were each treated with 3 to 6 tablets of zeolite (900mg. Each) every 3 hours.

In the second study, 72 volunteer patients with acute diarrhea were treated with the same dosage in the first study.

The third study was a comparative study in which diabetic patients with vascular impairments (neuropathic diarrhea) were either given a zeolite-based anti-medication or an anti-motility drug. Due to vascular impairments, recovery of patients must be achieved within 24 hours. The results revealed no significant difference. Further, the study demonstrated that a second dose of the zeolite-based anti-diarrheic medication had no adverse side effects, a benefit that the anti-motility drug could not boast.

In a fourth study, 435 volunteers with acute diarrhea resulting from food poisoning (the main cause of acute diarrhea in adults) were treated with the zeolite-based anti-diarrheic. 75 percent of the patients recovered from the diarrhea within 24 hours and the remaining 25 percent recovered during the following 12 hours.

Almost all the patients in the four studies showed good tolerance to treatment with the zeolite-based anti-diarrheic and none dropped out of the clinical trials due to side effects.

Rodriguez-Fuentes et al, 1997

Use of Zeolite in Various Canine Tumor Treatments

A study of the effects of using zeolite for various canine tumors were performed on 51 dogs. Before the treatment all the dogs received clinical examinations. Zeolite was given to the dogs orally, while affected skin areas were sprinkled with powder.

Mammary gland tumors were tested in 9 females between 6 and 15 years of age. The best results were noted in mammary adenocarcinoma. Smaller tumors disappeared after 3 weeks of taking zeolite, while larger tumors had reduced in size by half after 4 weeks.

Tumors of the skin and mucous membrane were tested in 9 dogs between 6 and 12 years of age. After receiving zeolite for a certain period of time, all formations disappeared, but reappeared after zeolite intake ceased. One week after taking zeolite was resumed the formation decreased in size once again.

Prostate tumors were tested in 6 dogs. Within one week of receiving zeolite symptoms had completely disappeared.

The influence of zeolite on lymphoma was tested on 9 dogs. All the dogs had perked up after receiving the preparation for 3 days, and after one week were behaving normally. Their blood count was normal one month later.

Lung tumors in 3 dogs had decreased in size by 50% after one month. Two dogs lived another year.

Bone cancer was diagnosed in 3 dogs and two of the dogs have been receiving zeolite for a year and a half.

With various other tumors, it was confirmed that in all dogs there was an improvement in overall condition.

Dr. Ljiljana Bedric Ph.D. Veterinary Medicine in Zagreb, Croatia

Author's Note: As of this writing, all clinical studies of zeolite have used the *powder* form.

Humic Acid

When the immune system is working properly, we remain healthy. However, the immune system can and does become compromised. This may be a result of incessant environmental assaults from exposure to pesticides (Agent Orange) and pollutants (Gulf War Syndrome) in the air, food and water, or poor nutrition as a contributing factor. When our bodies become overwhelmed, the regulatory features of the immune system weaken and become less effective, resulting in leaving the body susceptible to viruses such as: Epstein-Barr, Hepatitis, Herpes, Influenza and AIDS.

Viruses are very small. They are referred to as sub-cellular organism, meaning they are smaller than cells, smaller than bacteria and certainly smaller than most human host cells. Viruses are intracellular molecular parasites. They enter the body silently, and as in the cases of HIV and the different types of Hepatitis, they often do so without notice, using our cells to manufacture substances needed for their own replication and life cycle. They have no metabolic life of their own outside of host cell, which makes them dependent on living cells for their existence.

There are over 4000 known types of viruses, but less than 3 percent are well characterized, with new viruses being discovered regularly. Classification of viruses is based on several criteria, predominantly by the type of nucleic acid (DNA or RNA).

Among the DNA types are viruses that cause:

- chicken pox
- warts
- smallpox

- shingles
- hepatitis B
- common cold
- herpes simplex

Among the RNA types are viruses that cause:

- yellow fever
- polio
- hepatitis C
- rubella
- HIV
- measles
- bronchitis
- influenza
- encephalitis

There are three locations where viruses typically enter the human body: the respiratory tract (nose, throat and lungs); the gastrointestinal tract (mouth, stomach and intestines); and the genitourinary tract (the sex organs and urinary area). Viruses gain entry into the body via the respiratory tract through inhalation of air contaminated with the viruses people have expelled through coughing or sneezing; via the gastrointestinal tract through contaminated food, as in hepatitis A; via genitourinary tract through sexual intercourse as with HIV and herpes. In effect, the immune system receives a surprise attack and its response must be appropriately strong enough to eliminate the viruses. Often, as in HIV and HCV (Hepatitis C), there is no immediate immune response, as the virus has stealth mechanisms to outsmart the body's natural defenses.

Hope comes from great deposits of animal and plant material (humates) sealed away from wind and rain for millions of years, that have decomposed and then been compressed together by the million of tons of Earth above.

This process locks in their seventy-two nutrients. Humates are safe materials existing in all soils. They have been around since the beginning of time. Scientists have most appropriately referred to humic acid (which comes from humates) as the antiviral answer. One of the many reasons for the excitement involves the effect that humic acid has in its dramatic ability to penetrate even deadly ultra-microscopic viruses.

Viruses encapsulate themselves within an impenetrable protein barrier where defense mechanisms cannot reach them. Humic acid puts a coating around the viruses preventing them from adhering to healthy cells. It prevents the virus from reproducing. This is called *viral fusion inhibitors*. The viruses then become vulnerable to attack by the immune system, which is also strengthened by humic acid.

Benefits from a consistent long-term plan of dietary supplementation of humic acid are:

- Increasing resistance to colds and flu, infection and disease.
- Supercharging the immune system.
- Assisting in purging parasites, pathogens and viruses from the body.
- Restoring the body to its optimum potential over time.
- Creating an immediate feeling of well-being

Humic acid may help as a preventative and a curative for a broad range of viruses, which include:

- Influenza
- Common cold
- Herpes, oral, genital, shingles, Epstein-Barr
- Hepatitis A, B, C
- AIDS
- Warts (Human Papilloma Virus)
- West Nile
- Yellow Fever
- Hantavirus
- Gastroenteritis
- Cervical cancer

I have found ZEO Health's Zeolite-AV, to be an effective anti-viral and immune support supplement. The combination of very pure zeolite along with a potent and concentrated humic acid, to be responsible for alleviating many individuals' fight against chronic viruses.

Protocol for taking Zeolite:

- **Normal adult maintenance use:** two (2) capsules twice daily, or 5 grams zeolite powder once a day for at least 90 days.
- **Normal child maintenance use:** one (1) capsule twice daily, or 2 grams zeolite powder once a day for at least 90 days.
- **Normal adult detoxification use:** six (6) capsules two times a day or 5 grams zeolite powder twice a day
- **Normal child detoxification use:** three (3) capsules two times a day or 2 grams zeolite powder twice a day.

Cancer program and other related health issues:

- Six (6) capsules three times daily or 5 grams zeolite powder three times a day.
- **Diarrhea treatment program:** six (6) capsules or 5 grams zeolite powder with meals, as symptoms subside three (3) capsules twice daily or 2 grams zeolite powder twice a day.
- **Hangover treatment program:** six (6) capsules or 5 grams zeolite powder before drinking and/or six (6) capsules or 5 grams zeolite powder after 3 drinks.

Protocol for taking Zeolite with Humic Acid

- **Normal adult dosage:** two (2) capsules twice a day.
- **Normal child dosage:** one (1) capsule twice a day.
- For other needs, take four (4) capsules three times a day.

Note: Drink at least 8 glasses of water throughout the day to ensure adequate hydration.

Testimonials

"Love ZEO Health's products. I am a former MLM zeolite distributor. My upline there had told me that there is no way to tell in advance if the product is going to help someone or not. She told me they just have to try it and see. Some people it helps and some it doesn't, she said. An overweight nurse practitioner (NP)friend weighing 250 lbs. had bought the MLM drops from me and reported she noticed no effect at all from taking the entire contents of the dropper bottle as directed. A nutritionist friend who had sold a MLM zeolite product for years told me the NP would need to take at least twice the recommended dosage to notice an effect due to her weight. The nutritionist switched to ZEO Health and I did too. The NP just got your new micronized zeolite from me yesterday. She took one scoop full last night and this morning when she got up and voided her urine smelled very strongly of metal. She is excited about your product now. Your product must be much more effective than the competition! I sold your Zeolite Pure to a friend with knee achiness with stiffness and mild pain which she had for a number of years. It had improved in recent years due to improved diet. The discomfort completely vanished the second day after she started taking your zeolite pure product once a day".
All the best,
Nancy T. RN

"I just wanted to drop you a line about the mysterious ways zeolite has been working in my household. After you prescribed it, I read that it helps with Crohn's and Colitis. My cat has colitis. Not to get too graphic, but the poor thing has blood and mucus coming out when pooping. His stools are often very loose, and I find little poop drippings outside of the litter box and on the windowsill where he sits. (Sorry I know it's not pretty!) Anyway, I started mixing a little bit of the powder in with his morning wet food, and almost immediately noticed a HUGE difference. No more blood, mucus, or loose stools. Nearly all the little marks on the window sills are gone. I have noticed that if I forget to mix the zeolite powder in for a couple days, it will easily come

back. The vet suggested only expensive wet food as a solution, but it never helped and he was always hungry. I cannot believe how much zeolite alone has helped and I was able to get him back on his regular dry/wet food diet. Just wanted to let you know that it's not only helped me, but also my furry baby!" Forever grateful for this miracle powder!
Gina P.

"Doctors told me I have prostate cancer and metastates in some bones. I started hormone therapy. a friend of mine living in Canada sent me zeolite powder from ZEO Health.. I started zeolite also. after 6 months doctors (Hacettepe University, one of the biggest in turkey) told me my MRI seems good. No bad news about new metastases. after another 6 months no sign of metastases, and they asked me if I did some thing special. I said zeolite. They didn't care much. I used zeolite continuous one year. now its nearly 2018. I get hormone therapy from time to time and when hormone therapy starts, I start zeolite. and my doctors still don't ask me anything about zeolite. just say "..God is with you..so still you are alive."
Sincerely,
Guneş T.

"I have been using Zeolite Pure powder to help rid my system of toxins that have been causing the latest kidney issue called "Minimal Change Disease". The medical profession, after a painful kidney biopsy and loading me up with prescription drugs, and CT Scans, blood tests, UAs, etc… still has no clue what is causing the disease. So I started on a new diet of mostly fresh fruits, vegetables, beans, rice, some chicken, and taking zeolite and my Stage 3 kidney disease (GFR 53) improved to Stage 2 (GFR 79) within 4-5 weeks!

I would love to tell my story and help many others who have been diagnosed with "Minimal Change Disease" (or any other disease) to know how important it is to consider the impact toxins have on your immune system and how they can use the safest product that helps eliminate them, zeolite".
Chuck R.

"I did finally order from the link you gave me in U.K. and am feeling better taking my zeolite again♡ , my detoxification pathways are not working properly with this Heavy Metal Poisoning. I have MCS and leaky gut too so I had a lot of 'reabsorbtion' and/or 'retoxification' going on and I feel that the Zeolite is helping to prevent this as well. It relieves my MCS symptoms, especially severe 'crisis' on and after exposures, and I really noticed this when I ran out. Thanks again, ZEO Health"

Regards, *Therese*

"Your help and expertise, was invaluable to me. Helped many, many people. I myself, had heavy metal toxicity. I had testing done on myself, from several practitioners. With results, of metals, Mercury, lead etc. at very high levels. After taking zeolite powder, and being retested, my levels decreased substantially, to the point where, I have below levels of all metals. I with out a doubt, know that this product Zeolite Pure, has been the one thing that I will not do without. Proof that I have is my testing done at well know labs, and physicians, that are well respected, and well renowned in their expert fields. I will always be grateful, to you, for introducing me to Zeolite Pure by ZEO Health".

Best regards, *Elaine*

"I started out taking Zeolite -AV for HPV on my vocal chords. After six months it was gone(!) Two years later, I'm happy to report no recurrence of the virus during this time. Another happy coincidence, my husband had a skin condition called lychenplanus, which the dermatologist said was "manageable" but not curable. He started taking Zeolite -AV also, but at the rate of one capsule twice a day. I'm happy to report that after 8 weeks, the burning lychenplanus in his mouth resolved and after eight months, the thick, itchy, burny purple lychenplanus lesions on his legs have reduced to normal skin levels, the skin is flexible again, burning and itching have stopped and there is just mildly dark pigmentation where the lesions were. I believe if he had been willing to take more capsules each day, he would've had faster results. In any case, this is a release from purgatory for my husband"! THANK YOU!

Geraldine

"Recently, I came down with a very bad case of influenza. Normally this leads to severe respiratory distress. I was given Zeolite-AV to take every six hours. Within forty-eight hours all my symptoms were gone. I am very grateful for this product and I will continue to keep humic acid in my house for myself and my animals."
Meg C.

"For the last fifteen years I have lived with genital herpes. About once a month I would expect an outbreak. The medication I was taking was not helping. I began taking Zeolite-AV at the suggested dosage and the infection cleared up in a few days. I take a daily dose and I have not had a reoccurrence."
Denise Z

"A year ago I was diagnosed with hepatitis C. A friend suggested I start taking Zeolite-AV. I was tested again six weeks later and the results were negative. The doctors could not believe that the hepatitis C was gone. Thank you, thank you."
Gary D

"I have suffered for decades from IBS with diarrhea. I have never found a cure or treatment that worked. I was on dangerous prescription drugs for a period of time that gave me some relief, always aware of the symptoms of Ischemic bowel which could have killed me.

One day I was doing some research and found Esdifan. I ordered it out of curiosity and to my surprise, it worked! I continued to do more research to see what it was that made it so fabulous. It was Zeolite! I never go anywhere without my Esdifan and continue to use zeolite powders in my smoothies daily to pull out the heavy metals in my body. I would recommend everyone use zeolite powders daily to fight radiation, heavy metal, and toxins from our environment. I am a nurse working in anti-aging medicine. I love what I do and want to let everyone know how I have been helped by zeolite!
Joyce W.

Frequently Asked Questions about Zeolite

Q: *What is a zeolite?*

Zeolites are natural volcanic minerals that are mined in certain parts of the world. What makes zeolites so powerful, it's one of the few negatively charged minerals found in nature and zeolites have cage-like structure that allows space for large, positively charged ions to be attracted to it, then trapped and eliminated from the body. *Note,* not all mines are alike. There are different types with varying purity levels of zeolite at each mine throughout the world.

Q: *Can I take zeolite with other medications?*

As far as it is known, zeolite has no drug interactions and no side effects.

Q: *Is zeolite patented in the United States?*

There is a U.S. Patent on the powder form of zeolite for oral use, and there is a U.S. Patent on the liquid form for injectable use only.

Q: *How does it work?*

Zeolite has a chelation-like effect in removing heavy metals, pesticides, herbicides, and other positively charged toxins from the system. Zeolites negatively charged crystalline structure is what makes this possible. Its crystal act as 'cages', inside of which are positive ions. These positive ions switch places with positively charged toxins in the body. These toxins become tightly binded to the zeolite, which is eventually excreted from the body. The main benefit of binding toxins in this manner is they are 100 percent excreted.

Zeolite's binding power was proven during the Chernobyl disaster, when tons of it were used to remove radioactive cesium and strontium-90 before they contaminated local water symptoms. Acting primarily as a chelator, zeolite trapped these hazardous materials within its crystalline cage structure.

Q: *How long do I need to take a zeolite supplement?*

Normal protocol is 90 days, however for certain conditions, a longer period of time is suggested. Based on all of the health benefits of taking zeolite, this is a product that needs to be taken daily indefinitely, since we are exposed to toxins every day.

Q: *When taking zeolite internally, are there any heavy metals released in the body?*

I have found one of the purest zeolites (ZEO Health) and through various tests, that mimic stomach acids, there were no heavy metals released in the body with this powder form.

Q: *Will I go through a "healing crisis?"*

A healing crisis is when the body's natural defense systems are waging war on the illness itself and are trying to purge the illness from the body. People whose systems are quite toxic may go through a healing crisis. During this time, symptoms may worsen. However, this healing crisis will normally only last a few short days. When it is over, the body heals very rapidly. Improvements in health will be extremely noticeable. The healing crisis can be uncomfortable but once it has passed, people have been astounded at how well they begin to feel. In all cases, zeolite has produced positive results that have been observed in a time period ranging from a few days to as many as twelve weeks, normally averaging three to nine weeks. Unlike many other detoxifying products, zeolite seems to have a low or nonoccurrence of "health crisis" effects.

Q: *How can zeolite help the body's immune system combat different illnesses?*

Zeolite helps balance pH levels in your body, supports a healthy immune system and helps remove heavy metals and other cancer causing toxins from your body. Detoxification is the key foundation of staying healthy.

Q: Can I give this to my pets?

Yes. Zeolite is an excellent supplement to aid in detoxifying animals, especially if they have cancer.

Q: What is Humic Acid?

Humic acid has been discovered to be a significant miracle of nature. A part of the humate structure of enriched composing soil, it has been the subject of extensive scientific research, and is used now the world over as a dietary supplement to aid the body's ability to maintain overall health.

Q: How can Humic Acid help the body's immune system combat different illnesses?

All viruses must bind to host cells in order to reproduce. Humic acid has been shown in numerous vitro studies to block this process (including AIDS, Herpes, Influenza and Hemorrhagic Fever). The immune system then eliminates these viruses.

Q: Can I give this to my pets?

Yes. Humic acid is an excellent prevention for para-virus, a highly contagious disease for dogs, and West Nile virus in other pets and livestock animals.

Conclusion

Since 1997, scientists, doctors and medical researchers in Croatia, Austria, Germany and the United States have performed extensive studies that have confirmed the benefits of using zeolite in a wide variety of health applications. It is being researched just how zeolite may assist in the production of tumor suppressor cells and immune system helper cells, which are known to strengthen natural immunity. We are faced with a number of health challenges today. Zeolite is an exceptionally powerful antioxidant capable of cleansing the body of free radicals and heavy metals.

Medical studies show that difficult respiratory illnesses are readily resolved with humic acid dietary supplementation. Humic acid has the power to protect against cancer and tumors using special humic substance therapies. Combining humic acid (with it's viral fusion inhibitor) and zeolite (powder), synergestically make a perfect way to create homeostasis in the body.

Resource Directory

Zeolite supplements are available in a variety of forms; however, not every form provides optimal benefit.

Below are the sources I highly recommend:

ZEO Health
www.zeohealth.com
(845) 353-5185

Regal Supplements
www.regalsupplements.com
(845) 536-5511

www.zeolitedosing.com

www.zeolitetestimonials.com

References

Breck, D.W., "Crystalline molecular sieves," *Journal Chem. Edu.* 41:678-679 (1964)

Colella, C. "Natural zeolites in environmentally friendly process and application", *Stud. Surface Science Catalysis* 125:641-655 (1999)

Garces, J.M. "Observations on zeolite applications," Proceedings of the 12th International Conference on Zeolites Material Research Society, *Warrendale* 551-566 (1999)

Mirvish, S.S., "Etiology of gastric cancer, introgastric, nitrosamide formation and other theories", *Journal National Cancer Institute* Vol. 71, 629-647 (1983)

Mumpton, F.A., "Natural Zeolites," *Westview Press Inc.,* 33-44 (1984)

Peiper, H., "The Secrets of Staying Young", Safe Goods Publishing (1994)

Ramos, A.J., Fin k-Gremmels, J. and Hernandez, E., "Prevention of toxic effects of mycotoxins by means of nonnutritive adsorbent compounds," *Journal of Food Protection* Vol. 59, 631-641 (1996)

Rapp, D., *Our Toxic World,* EMRF Publ. (2004)

Rodriguez-Fuentes, G., Barrios, M.A., "Enterex-antidiarrheic drug based on purified natural clinoptilolite," *Zeolites* 19:441-448 (1997)

Wang, Y., Zhu, J.H., Yan, D. Huang, W.Y., "Adsorption of N-nitrosamines by zeolites in solutions," *Stud. Surf. Sci. Catal.* 135, 226 (2001)

Weiner, H.C., "Oral tolerance: immune mechanisms and treatment of autoimmune diseases," *Immunology Today* Vol. 18, 335-343

Zhu, J.H., "Attempt to adsorb N-nitrosamines in solution by use of zeolites," *Chemosphere* 44, 949-956 (2001)

About The Author

Dr. Howard Peiper is a Doctor of Naturopathic Medicine. In 1972, he received his degree in Naturopathy. After a decade in private practice, Dr. Peiper became a successful consultant, speaker and writer.

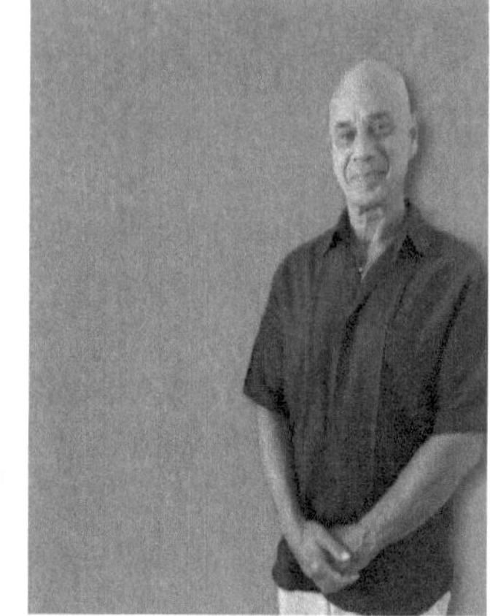

Throughout the years, his cutting-edge articles appeared in numerous medical journals and magazines. He also serves on the medical advisory board for several nutritional companies.

Dr. Peiper has written several bestselling titles, including: *The A.D.D. and A.D.H.D. Diet*, The *Secrets to Staying Young* and *New Hope for Serious Diseases*. He is a frequent guest speaker on radio and television programs. He even hosted his own shows, including the award-winning television show, "Partners in Healing."

NOTES:

NOTES: